CARDIOLOGY RESEARCH AND CLINICAL DEVELOPMENTS

# CLOPIDOGREL RESPONSE IN ACUTE CORONARY SYNDROME: CLINICAL IMPLICATIONS AND EMERGING THERAPIES

# CARDIOLOGY RESEARCH AND CLINICAL DEVELOPMENTS

Additional books in this series can be found on Nova's website
under the Series tab.

Additional E-books in this series can be found on Nova's website
under the E-book tab.

CARDIOLOGY RESEARCH AND CLINICAL DEVELOPMENTS

# CLOPIDOGREL RESPONSE IN ACUTE CORONARY SYNDROME: CLINICAL IMPLICATIONS AND EMERGING THERAPIES

ANTONIO DE MIGUEL CASTRO
ALEJANDRO DIEGO NIETO
JUAN CARLOS CUELLAS RAMÓN
ARMANDO PÉREZ DE PRADO
JAVIER GUALIS CARDONA
AND
FELIPE FÉRNANDEZ-VÁZQUEZ

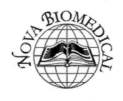

**Nova Biomedical Books**
*New York*

## Library of Congress Cataloging-in-Publication Data

Clopidogrel response in acute coronary syndrome : clinical implications and emerging therapies / Antonio de Miguel Castro ... [et al.].
   p. ; cm.
 Includes bibliographical references and index.
  ISBN 978-1-61761-585-6 (softcover)
  1. Clopidogrel. 2. Coronary heart disease--Chemotherapy. I. Miguel Castro, Antonio de.
  [DNLM: 1. Acute Coronary Syndrome--drug therapy. 2. Platelet Aggregation Inhibitors--therapeutic use. 3. Ticlopidine--pharmacology. 4. Ticlopidine--therapeutic use. WG 300]
  RC685.C6C575 2010
  616.1'23061--dc22
                         2010031178

*Published by Nova Science Publishers, Inc. † New York*

# Contents

# Preface

The benefits of clopidogrel on the treatment of acute coronary syndromes are well established. However, not all patients respond in the same way to clopidogrel therapy, and there are patients who suffer major adverse cardiovascular events despite being on treatment, emerging the concept of clopidogrel resistance. This chapter is focused on this topic, mainly in the definition, response assessment, clinical implications, patients' management and emerging therapies (prasugrel, cangrelor and ticagrelor).

There is an interindividual variability in response to clopidogrel therapy, and lower response has been correlated with recurrent adverse cardiovascular events, including late stent thrombosis. Nevertheless, there is not clear and consensual definition of clopidogrel resistance. Clopidogrel response follows a normal distribution, so it would be more appropriate to refer to as variable response to clopidogrel rather than clopidogrel resistance, with its clinical implications: the lower response, the higher probability of suffering thrombotic events. Due to the misleading definition of "resistance" and non-standardized method to assess platelet inhibition, current guidelines do not routinely recommend the use of platelet function assays to monitor the inhibitory effect of antiplatelet drugs and guide therapies. Clopidogrel loading doses higher than 300 mg and daily maintenance doses higher than 75 mg are not routinely recommended by current guidelines, although 600 mg clopidogrel loading dose seems to be safe and effective, and could be used when a faster onset of action is required. Unfortunately, the management of patients with low response to clopidogrel remains uncertain. Strict control of risk factors may improve clopidogrel response. Recently, emerging therapies such as prasugrel and ticagrelor have shown better results than clopidogrel in the prevention of death from cardiovascular cause, nonfatal myocardial infarction, or stroke, but at expenses of a higher rate of bleeding events. It remains uncertain whether patients who suffer a thrombotic event being on clopidogrel treatment would benefit from switching to prasugrel or ticagrelor therapy.

# Abbreviations List

| | |
|---|---|
| ACS | Acute Coronary Syndrome |
| ADP | Adenosine Diphosphate |
| AMI | Acute Myocardial Infarction |
| DES | Drug Eluting Stents |
| MACE | Major Adverse Cardiovascular Event |
| IPA | Inhibition of Platelet Aggregation |
| NSTE-ACS | Non-ST-segment Elevation Acute Coronary Syndrome |
| PCI | Percutaneous Coronary Intervention |
| PRU | Platelet Reaction Unit |
| STEMI | ST Elevation Myocardial Infarction |
| VASP | Vasodilator Stimulated Phosphoprotein |

# Introduction

Platelets play a central role in the pathogenesis of acute coronary syndromes (ACS) and complications after percutaneous coronary interventions (PCI). Rupture or erosion of atherosclerotic lesions facilitates the interaction of flowing blood with the inner components of the atherosclerotic lesions. Tissue factor in the plaque activates the clotting cascade leading to acute thrombus formation with its clinical manifestations: unstable angina, non-ST segment elevation acute coronary syndrome (NSTE-ACS), ST elevation myocardial infarction (STEMI) and sudden cardiac death [1, 2].

The benefits of antiplatelet therapy for the treatment and prevention of acute coronary events clinically support the role of platelets in the pathogenesis of atherothrombotic process. The most commonly used antiplatelet drugs are aspirin and clopidogrel, alone or in combination.

Clopidogrel is a second-generation thienopyridine that selective and irreversibly blocks the P2Y12-adenosine diphosphate (ADP) receptor[3, 4]. Despite their platelet inhibitory effects, both aspirin and clopidogrel monotherapy are considered a safe although weak therapy. Given their different mechanisms of action, coadministration of both antiplatelet agents attains higher platelet inhibition [5]. Several clinical trials have demonstrated the additional beneficial role of clopidogrel in addition to aspirin to prevent stent thrombosis after PCI [6-8] and the reduction in the incidence of major adverse cardiovascular events (MACE) in patients with NSTE-ACS [9] and STEMI [10-12]. Nevertheless, dual antiplatelet therapy is not recommended for the prevention of atherothrombotic events in patients with stable cardiovascular disease or multiple cardiovascular risk factors [13].

However, not all individuals show the same response to clopidogrel treatment, and there are patients who suffer adverse events despite being on treatment. Variable response to clopidogrel treatment has been described extensively in different clinical settings and the term of clopidogrel resistance has arisen, but this term is misleading and a standard definition is still lacking; in addition, regardless of the different mechanisms of platelet inhibition, poor responsiveness to aspirin has also been associated with lower response to clopidogrel [14].

This chapter is focused on this topic, mainly in the definition, response assessment, clinical implications, patients' management and emerging therapies (prasugrel, cangrelor and ticagrelor).

# Chapter I

# Resistance/Variable Response to Clopidogrel. Does it Exist?

There is no standardized definition of clopidogrel resistance, and the exact prevalence remains uncertain; ranges from 5 to 44% [14-22] have been reported in different studies. Resistance definition can be based on a clinical or biochemical approach.

The clinical definition of resistance is based on the failure to prevent adverse events in patients "on treatment". There is large evidence supporting that low response to antiplatelet agents correlates with adverse events, but given the multifactorial etiopathogenesis of atherothrombotic events, results inaccurate to define clopidogrel resistance based on the recurrence of adverse events. Under these clinical criteria, the term "clinical resistance" should be avoided and it would more appropriate to use the term "treatment failure".

The biochemical definition of resistance is based on the failure to achieve "adequate" inhibitory standards on laboratory tests of platelet function. The inhibitory effect has been determined as absolute difference between pre- and post-treatment platelet reactivity (PPR) or percent reduction in aggregation parameters obtained at baseline and after treatment; the latter methodology is also termed IPA (inhibition of platelet aggregation). Patients' response to clopidogrel follows a typical normal distribution (something common to almost all drugs). Therefore, response to clopidogrel therapy shouldn't be considered in a dichotomic way (YES/NO response), but a continuous variable. According to the normal (bell-shaped) curve of response to clopidogrel treatment, it is expectable to find ≈5% of hyper- and hypo-responders, as it is expectable with any other drug [23]. The magnitude of (low) response to clopidogrel treatment might be dynamic, varying even over time during long-term treatments. More importantly, the cut-off values are arbitrary and vary among studies, so it would be more appropriate to refer to as variable response rather than resistance to clopidogrel.

Some studies [24-30] support that *post-treatment platelet reactivity* is a better estimate of thrombotic risk than the degree of IPA, since IPA (percent decrease in platelet aggregation values) does not take into account the absolute level of platelet reactivity. This becomes even more confusing when Gurbel et al [15] showed that there are patients with low post-treatment platelet reactivity who are clopidogrel non-responders (defined as a percent decrease in aggregation values) and some patients who are clopidogrel responders continue to have high post-treatment platelet reactivity.

The biochemical definition of resistance or variable response to clopidogrel (according to laboratory test) has several limitations: different assays used for platelet function assessment (every one with its own limitations), usage of diverse agonist (and doses) to induce and measure platelet aggregation, variable cut-off values, and different time window chosen to measure the platelet aggregation.

Furthermore, the impact of laboratory estimation of response to any antiplatelet therapy is not completely understood, since the relationship between resistance/variable response and adverse clinical events is very heterogeneous. Similarly to clopidogrel resistance, the term aspirin resistance has also arisen, and the results of a recent meta-analysis [31] are very illustrative because stand out the significant different aspirin resistance prevalence depending on the platelet function assay used: 6% vs 26% with optical aggregometry and point-of-care tests, respectively, showing the difficulty to establish a standardized definition of resistance and method to assess platelet inhibition. The correlation between platelet function test and adverse events have been established in different clinical settings with diverse inclusion criteria, clinical end points and follow-up, different clopidogrel loading/maintenance dosage and, more importantly, in small size clinical trials with limited number of cardiovascular events.

The optimal level of inhibition of platelet aggregation to prevent cardiovascular events may vary upon the clinical situation and, to date, there are no universally accepted IPA and/or post-treatment platelet reactivity thresholds identifying patients at higher risk for adverse events in specific clinical settings. Ongoing trials are currently evaluating whether targeting a particular degree of platelet inhibition, either with novel antiplatelet agents or higher doses of current drugs, will prove to be safe and efficacious. These studies will provide the critical missing information about the capability of these methods for monitoring antiplatelet therapies in cardiac patients and other clinical scenarios. Due to the misleading definition of "resistance" and non-standardized method to assess platelet inhibition, current guidelines do not routinely recommend the use of platelet function assays to monitor the inhibitory effect of antiplatelet drugs and guide therapies [32-34].

Another important factor to take into account when analyzing the degree of PPR and IPA achieved with any antiplatelet treatment, is the practical impossibility of obtaining the real baseline values (pre-treatment) of platelet reactivity in some specific clinical settings, since certain pathological conditions such as ACS are characterized by ongoing thrombosis resulting in increased platelet reactivity, leading to unknow the baseline platelet reactivity prior to the ongoing ACS.

# Chapter II

# Mechanisms of Variable Response to Clopidogrel

Interindividual variable response to clopidogrel is multifactorial and the mechanisms have not been fully elucidated; these mechanism can be divided into pharmacokinetic (failure to achieve/maintain adequate levels of the active drug) or pharmacodynamic factors (despite adequate levels there is a failure to inhibit the specific receptors). Also the clinical, environmental, cellular and genetic factors play a role in this regard. Potential mechanisms of variable response to clopidogrel are summarized in table 1.

Increased (baseline) platelet activity and thrombotic burden in specific clinical settings (ACS, diabetes, dyslipemia, heart failure, PCI, and obesity) may also contribute to "lower response" to antiplatelet therapies. Clopidogrel exerts their inhibitory effect via one of the several pathways triggering platelet activation and aggregation. In addition, clopidogrel does not abolish platelet response to stronger agonist such as thrombin, epinephrine and collagen. In high-risk clinical situations, such as ACS, characterized by a high thrombin generation environment, a higher platelet inhibition might be required to protect against atherothrombotic events. However, there are clinical trials involving non-STEMI [35] and STEMI patients [36] that have shown that a dramatically higher inhibition of platelet aggregation achieved with glycoprotein IIb/IIIa inhibitors is not always followed by clinical benefits.

**Table 1. Potential Mechanism of Variable Response to Clopidogrel**

| |
|---|
| 1. Reduced clopidogrel bioavailability |
| - Non-compliance to clopidogrel therapy |
| - Under-dosing or inappropriate dosing of clopidogrel |
| - Poor absorption |
| - Drug-drug interactions involving cytochrome P450 |
| 2. Genetic variables: |
| - Polymorphism of $P2Y_{12}$ |
| - Polymorphism of cytochrome P450 |
| - Polymorphism of multidrug resistance transporter |
| - Polymorphism of GP Ia |
| - Polymorphism of GP IIb/IIIa |
| 3. Increased release of ADP |
| 4. Increased $P2Y_{12}$ receptors |
| 5. Clinical factors leading to high pre-treatment platelet reactivity: |
| - Acute coronary syndrome |
| - Diabetes mellitus/Insulin resistance |
| - Elevated body mass index |
| 6. Up-regulation of $P2Y_{12}$ independent pathways |
| 7. Up-regulation of P2Y independent pathways: |
| - Thrombin |
| - Thromboxane $A_2$ |
| - Collagen |
| - Epinephrine |
| 8. Increased turn-over of platelets |

ADP= Adenosine Diphosphate; GP= Glycoprotein.

# Genetic Polymorphism

After intestinal absorption, clopidogrel is a prodrug that needs hepatic metabolism to the generation of its active metabolite (85% is hydrolyzed by esterases in the blood). Specifically, 2 sequential oxidative steps through the cytochrome P450 (CYP) system are needed. A variety of P450 enzymes contribute to clopidogrel metabolism. The first metabolic step, which leads to 2-oxo-clopidogrel, is dependent on 3 enzymes (CYP1A2, CYP2B6, and CYP2C19), whereas the second step, which culminates in the active metabolite, involves 4 enzymes (CYP2B6, CYP2C9, CYP2C19, and CYP3A4). Pharmacogenetic studies have studied different genes polymorphisms implicated in the pharmacokinetics and pharmacodynamics of clopidogrel. Among these, genes included encode proteins and enzymes involved in intestinal absorption, hepatic metabolism, and platelet membrane receptors.

There are consistent data that relate clopidogrel variability response to hepatic CYP polymorphisms, mainly, the CYP2C19 loss of function polymorphism [37]. Importantly, in addition to modulation of pharmacodynamic and pharmacokinetic profiles, this polymorphism has also been associated with greater ischemic event rates [38], including stent thrombosis [39]. These findings have led to suggest genetic testing for this polymorphism as a screening measure for clopidogrel response. Point-of-care assays are currently under development to allow rapid genetic testing for this polymorphism.

# Drug-Drug Interactions

Another factor affecting response to clopidogrel is the possibility of drug-drug interactions (cardiac patients are being prescribed with multiple drugs). As previously described, clopidogrel is an inactive prodrug that requires two-step oxidation by the hepatic CYP system to generate its active compound. Drugs that are substrates or inhibit the CYP system can potentially interfere with the conversion of clopidogrel into its active metabolite, leading to reduce its antiplatelet effects. Among these drugs, there has been special focus on statins, proton pump inhibitors (PPIs) and calcium channel blockers, common concomitant drugs prescribed with clopidogrel in cardiac patients.

## Statins

Preliminary studies have shown that lipophilic statins, such as atorvastatin, lovastatin and simvastatin, which require CYP3A4 metabolization, hamper clopidogrel-induced antiplatelet effects [40, 41]. However, recent reports have denied this interaction [42, 43].

## Proton Pump Inhibitors

Patients receiving dual antiplatelet treatment with aspirin and clopidogrel are commonly treated with PPIs with the objective of minimising the risk of gastrointestinal (GI) bleeding complications. Current guidelines recommend prescription of a PPI in all patients under dual antiplatelet treatment [44]. Hepatic metabolization of PPIs is CYP-dependent and it has been hypothesized that a potential drug-drug interaction at the level of the hepatic CYP system exists causing an attenuated response to clopidogrel under concomitant omeprazole treatment due to diminished CYP-dependent metabolization of clopidogrel into its active thiol metabolite.

In a double-blind, placebo-controlled trial [45], 124 consecutive patients undergoing PCI treated with aspirin (75 mg/day) and clopidogrel (300 mg loading dose, followed by 75 mg/day) were randomized to receive omeprazole (20 mg/day) or placebo for 7 days. Clopidogrel effect was tested on days 1 and 7 in both groups by measuring vasodilator stimulated phosphoprotein (VASP) phosphorylation, expressed as platelet reactivity index (PRI). On Day 7, 16 patients (26.7%) were poor responders in the placebo group compared with 39 patients (60.9%) in the omeprazole group (p < 0.0001). The odds ratio of being a poor responder to clopidogrel when concomitantly treated with omeprazole was 4.31 (95%, CI 2.0 to 9.2). The clinical impact of these results was not assessed.

Different studies [46, 47] have confirmed the attenuating effects on clopidogrel response reported in the OCLA trial for the PPI omeprazole, but not for pantoprazole and esomeprazole, which do not attenuate the antiplatelet action of clopidogrel, supporting that the attenuating effects of PPI treatment on clopidogrel response are not a phenomenon observed for all PPIs in general. However, the results of the Clopidogrel Medco Outcomes study including 16.690 patients presented in the SCAI 2009 Annual Scientific Sessions (Las Vegas, Nevada, USA) defended a possible "class effect" for PPIs on top of clopidogrel therapy.

Several retrospective studies have evaluated the risk of adverse events associated with concomitant use of clopidogrel and PPIs. In patients undergoing PCI with DES, the prescription of a PPI at discharge was associated with a greater rate of MACE at 1 year, with an adjusted hazard ratio of 1.8 (95% confidence interval 1.1 to 2.7, p = 0.01) after multivariate analysis [48]. An additional study [49] has shown in patients after ACS that the use of clopidogrel plus PPIs is associated with an increased risk of death or rehospitalization for ACS compared with the use of clopidogrel without PPI (adjusted OR, 1.25; 95% CI, 1.11-1.41).

Great expectation was focus on the results of the COGENT trial, a large randomized double-blind, clinical trial. The COGENT trial was prematurely stopped with only 3627 patients enrolled out of the roughly 5000 investigators had expected to recruit. Patients requiring clopidogrel for at least 12 months (typically following NSTE-ACS, STEMI, or stent implantation) were included and randomized to receive omeprazole or placebo. The results of the COGENT trial were presented in the TCT 2009 Congress, San Francisco, California, USA, reporting (survival data out to 390 days) 67 cardiovascular events in the placebo group and 69 in the omeprazole group, with similar event curves (a composite of CV death, nonfatal AMI, CABG or PCI, or ischemic stroke). For the end points of MI alone and revascularization procedures alone, event curves once again were identical. In analyses taking into account baseline variables or medical history, there was no signal of increased cardiovascular events for patients treated with omeprazole in any subgroup. By contrast, looking just at GI events (upper-GI bleeding, symptomatic upper-GI bleeding, pain of presumed GI origin with underlying multiple erosive disease), researchers found that event rates were significantly higher in patients randomized to placebo.

Considering all available evidence, experts recommend that PPI use should be limited to situations clearly indicated in patients on clopidogrel treatment after PCI or ACS.

## Calcium-Channel Blockers

Calcium-channel blockers (CCBs) inhibit the cytochrome P450-3A4 enzyme, which metabolises clopidogrel to its active form. Two observational prospective studies have described the influence of CCBs on clopidogrel mediated platelet inhibition in vivo [50, 51]. In both studies, concomitant CCB therapy was significantly associated with decreased platelet inhibition by clopidogrel. Moreover, intake of CCBs was associated with adverse clinical outcomes, driven by a higher rate of revascularization procedures. Due to the small sample size, baseline differences between treatment groups and the observational nature instead of interventional of these studies, large randomized clinical trials are required before drawing definitive conclusions.

# Chapter III

# Is it Possible to Accurately Assess the Inhibitory Effect of Antiplatelt Drugs?

When assessing the inhibitory effect of any antiplatelet agent, the mechanism of action of the drug should be fully understood. It has been already noted that clopidogrel blocks the P2Y12-ADP receptor. Therefore, in order to assess the inhibitory effects of clopidogrel, an ADP-dependent technique should be respectively applied.

The different options to assess the inhibitory effect of clopidogrel have been described elsewhere [3, 52]; however, there is not standardized method and none of them evaluate platelet activation as a whole, since platelets can be activated by several different pathways. Table 2 summarizes the advantages and limitations of the more common asssays used to evaluate the response to clopidogrel.

Optical aggregometry is considered the gold standard to assess platelet activity, mainly because the abundance of data generated with this technique rather than its advantage over other techniques. Several circumstances as the time, equipment and training required for mastering it, makes this technique impracticable for the cath lab or private office daily practice. Therefore, several point-of-care devices have been developed to surpass the inconvenients of optical aggregomctry. Some of them have been specifically modified for assessing clopidogrel response.

The VerifyNow system (Accumetrics, San Diego, California, USA) is a point-of-care device that uses the same principle than platelet aggregometry but measures agglutination of fibrinogen-coated beads in whole blood in response to ADP and prostaglandin E1 in case of clopidogrel assay.

The Platelet Function Assay-100 (PFA-100) is a point-of-care device that simulates haemostasis by flowing whole blood through a cartridge that contains an aperture coated with collagen, epinephrine or ADP and the time required for aperture closure and cessation of blood flow is used as a measure of platelet activation.

**Table 2. Platelet Function Asssays to Evaluate Response to Clopidogrel**

| Laboratory Test | Advantages | Limitations |
|---|---|---|
| Optical aggregometry | Widely available Correlated with clinical outcomes Considered gold-standard | Poor reproducibility, operator- and interpreter-dependent Not specfic Uncertain sensitivity High sample volume and sample preparation Requirement for a skilled technician Length of assay time and labour intensive Assesses platelet function in the absence of erythrocytes and blood flow (shear stress) |
| Platelet Function Assay-100 | Point-of-care use Simplicity and rapidity Low sample volume Whole blood and no sample preparation Correlated with clinical outcomes | Uncertain specificity Uncertain sensitivity Expensive Not recommended for monitoring clopidogrel therapy Dependent on von Willebrand factor levels, citrate concentration haematocrit |
| VerifyNow Rapid Platelet Function Assay | Point-of-care use Simplicity and rapidity Low sample volume Whole blood and no sample preparation Correlated with clinical outcomes | Uncertain specificity Uncertain sensitivity Expensive |
| VASP Phosphorylation Assay | $P2Y_{12}$ receptor reactivity specific marker Low sample volume Whole blood | Specific assay for clopidogrel-induced platelet inhibition Flow cytometry requirement Requirement for a skilled technician Sample preparation Expensive Correlation with clinical outcomes less stablished |

VASP= Vasodilatador Stimulated Phosphoprotein.

The Multiplate analyzer (Dynabyte, Munich, Germany) is point-of-care device available for rapid and standardised assessment of platelet function parameters in different clinical settings. This device, based on multiple electrode platelet aggregometry, is highly capable of detecting the effect of clopidogrel treatment and the results correlate well with light transmission aggregometry.

Flow cytometry assessment of VASP phosphorilation assay (BioCytex, Marseilles, France) is a specific marker of P2Y12 receptor reactivity and, therefore, clopidogrel-induced inhibition, but this method is expensive and needs sample preparation, requires a flow cytometry and an experienced technician.

There are other laboratory test such as the point-of-care systems Plateletworks (Helena Laboratories, Beaumont, Texas, USA), Thromboelastography platelet mapping system (Haemoscope, Niles, Illinois, USA), and Impact cone and plate analyzer (DiaMed, Cressier, Switzerland) and flow cytometry to measure activation dependent changes in platelet surface P-selectin, platelet surface glycoprotein IIb/IIIa or leukocyte-platelet aggregates; however, these platelet function test are less studied than those described above and have not been tested in clinical settings to predict clinical outcomes; moreover, flow cytometry is too laborious to perform on a patient-to-patient basis.

From the practical point of view, it could be summarized that there are several alternatives for assessing resistance/variable response to clopidogrel. Despite the more friendly-use and speed of the point-of care devices, optical aggregometry and flow cytometry are still considered the best methodologies for accurately assessing platelet reactivity.

*Chapter IV*

# Clinical Implications of Variable Response to Clopidogrel

The clinical implications of low inhibition after clopidogrel therapy have been described in several clinical studies. Geisler et al [53] described a higher risk of cardiovascular events among "clopidogrel low-responders" compared to "clopidogrel normo-responders" in patients undergoing elective PCI. Similarly, Matetzky et al [16] showed that, in patients with AMI undergoing primary angioplasty, lower platelet inhibition at days 3 and 6 after PCI was associated with recurrent cardiovascular events at 6 months. Patients with stable angina (n=105) undergoing elective PCI, the only 2 cases of subacute stent thrombosis occurred among clopidogrel non-responders [17].

The prognostic value of post-treatment platelet reactivity has been correlated with clinical outcomes in different clinical trials, most of them involving a reduced number of patients with equally low number of events. In the POPULAR study [54] was evaluated the ability of multiple platelet function tests in predicting atherothrombotic events, including stent thrombosis, in clopidogrel pre-treated patients undergoing PCI with stent implantation. High PPR, when assessed by light transmittance aggregometry (both 5 µmol/L and 20 µmol/L ADP), VerifyNow P2Y12 assay, and Plateletworks, was significantly associated with atherothrombotic events. In contrast, the shear stress-based tests IMPACT-R (with and without ADP prestimulation) and the Dade PFA-100 system (the collagen/ADP and Innovance PFA P2Y) did not show an association with outcome. However, the predictability of these 3 tests was only modest. Cuisset et al [55] described that higher PPR is associated with higher incidence of myonecrosis after stenting for NSTE-ACS. Our group has shown that in patients with NSTEACS undergoing elective early PCI, PPR predicts myocardial damage better than response to clopidogrel [56]. Marcucci et al [57] showed that high PPR affects the severity of myocardial infarction independently of other clinical, procedural, and laboratory parameters in patients with AMI undergoing PCI.

A lot of expectancy was generated by two large clinical studies. Gurbel et al [58] demonstrated that PPR is higher in patients who suffered subacute stent thrombosis compared to those without thrombosis. The difference between both groups was significant, but a careful analysis of the data shows a significant overlapping on the individual data of platelet aggregation and/or thromboelastography from both groups. This overlapping significantly reduces the value of these methodologies when applied to a single patient debilitating their possibilities for individualized medicine. Similar data were reported by Hochholzer et al [24] in patients following elective PCI after 600 mg clopidogrel loading-dose: a 10% increase in ADP-induced platelet aggregation on treatment before PCI was associated with higher risk for 30-days events; in addition to the association between PPR and the risk for 30 days adverse events observed in this study, it should be noticeably marked that the same patients also shared the shortest time from clopidogrel loading dose to PCI (mean 1.8; range 0.8-4.0 hours); this observation is of critical importance on the basis of previous reports suggesting a minimum time of 4 to 6 hours for achieving the maximal antiplatelet effect of clopidogrel.

As previously noticed, PPR is considered a better estimate of thrombotic risk than the degree of IPA, since IPA (percent decrease in platelet aggregation values) does not take into account the absolute level of platelet reactivity. Our group published [30] that in patients with NSTE-ACS undergoing early coronary angiography, the independent predictors of MACE at 1 year were only PPR (10-unit increase in PPR is associated with adjusted OR [AOR], 1.12; 95% CI, 1.01-1.24; P=0.02) and previous antiplatelet therapy (AOR, 4.56; 95% CI, 1.13-23; P=0.033). Cuisset et al [25] described the relationship between PPR before PCI with the subsequent occurrence of MACE at 30-days follow-up in NSTE-ACS patients: irrespective of clopidogrel loading dose (300 mg vs 600 mg), only the persistence of high PPR was significantly associated with cardiovascular events, remarking the importance of the effect of antiplatelet treatment rather than the loading dose. In addition, it is also known that low platelet reactivity at the time of PCI, irrespective of whether this is due to pharmacological inhibition or low baseline platelet reactivity, is beneficial in terms of clinical outcomes [24]. Despite the number of patient enrolled in these studies, the still limited number of events hampers the validity of the conclusions.

# Drug Eluting Stent

Recent meta-analysis have associated drug-eluting stents (DES) with an increased risk of late stent thrombosis and adverse events compared to bare metal stents [59, 60]. A multivariate analysis has identified premature discontinuation of combined antiplatelet therapy as the major independent predictor for late stent thrombosis after DES deployment [61]. In fact, some studies have suggested an increase in the risk of stent thrombosis within drug eluting stents when clopidogrel is discontinued within 6 months after implantation by a factor of more than 30, and an increase by a factor of approximately 6 when clopidogrel is discontinued at 6 months or beyond [61, 62]. Lower response to antiplatelet therapy is also associated with an increased risk of late stent thrombosis in patients receiving DES [63, 64], more evident in patients with dual aspirin and clopidogrel non-responsiveness compared to isolated aspirin or clopidogrel non-responsiveness [65]. Of notice, different observational studies has suggested that early, but not late stent thrombosis, is influenced by residual platelet aggregation in patients treated with dual antiplatelet therapy undergoing PCI [66, 67]. Acute resistance/low response to antiplatelet therapy should not be a key factor since the definition of late stent thrombosis involves a minimum of 1-month post-stenting and very late stent thrombosis 12-months post-stenting. Therefore, DES late and very late stent thrombosis seems to be more correlated with early withdrawal rather to treatment failure. As such, prolonged dual-antiplatelet inhibition therapy for at least 1 year in patients with DES has been recommended. Any elective procedures with significant risk of bleeding should be deferred until appropriate completion of dual antiplatelet therapy [68]. In case of mandatory discontinuation, clopidogrel should be restarted as soon as possible.

A recent study by Park et al has reported that the use of dual antiplatelet therapy for a period longer than 12 months in patients who had received drug-eluting stents was not significantly more effective than aspirin monotherapy in reducing the rate of myocardial infarction or death from cardiac causes [69], but this finding has not been confirmed or refuted yet. Hence, larger, randomized clinical trials evaluating specifically the appropriate duration of dual antiplatelet therapy are needed.

# Chapter V

# What to do with Patients with Reduced Response to Clopidogrel Therapy?

Unfortunately, the management of patients with low response to clopidogrel remains uncertain. In an initial approach, certain factors such as patient compliance and appropriate dosage are assumed to take place. In addition, strict control of risk factors may improve the response to clopidogrel.

Inhibitory effects of clopidogrel are time- and dose-dependent; 600 mg loading dose of clopidogrel causes an earlier, more sustained and stronger inhibition of ADP-induced platelet aggregation than 300 mg loading dose [70, 71]. In addition, there is evidence that 600 mg loading dose of clopidogrel reduces recurrent atherothrombotic events without increasing major bleeding complications in patients undergoing elective PCI compared to 300 mg loading-dose [25, 72]. However, 900 mg clopidogrel loading dose does not result in further suppression of ADP-platelet aggregation, and the clinical impact of clopidogrel loading doses higher than 600 mg is not well established [73, 74]. In patients following elective PCI, at least 6 hours are necessary to achieve full antiplatelet effect after 300 mg clopidogrel loading-dose [74] and 2 hours after 600 mg loading-dose [24]. NSTE-ACS and PCI guidelines [32-34] do not support the routinely use of clopidogrel loading doses higher than 300 mg, and only when is necessary to achieve a more rapid onset of platelet inhibition, 600 mg clopidogrel loading dose may be used in STEMI patients following primary PCI as suggested by STEMI guidelines [75, 76].

The results of the ARMYDA-4 and ARMYDA-5 trials were presented in the TCT 2007 Scientific Sessions (Washington, Washington State, USA). The ARMYDA-4 (ARMYDA-RELOAD) trial assessed the additional clinical benefit of 600 mg clopidogrel loading dose pre-PCI compared to placebo in patients already on chronic clopidogrel treatment undergoing elective PCI in a prospective, randomized, double blind-design study (180 patients received clopidogrel and 180 patients placebo). No clinical benefit (composite end point of death, AMI and target vessel revascularization) was found at 30 days follow-up with the additional 600 mg clopidogrel loading. The ARMYDA-5 (ARMYDA-PRELOAD) trial evaluated the occurrence of clinical events (composite end point of death, AMI and target vessel revascularization) at 30 days follow-up in patients undergoing elective PCI receiving 600 mg clopidogrel loading dose 4-8 hours before PCI compared to 600 mg clopidogrel loading dose immediately before PCI. No clinical benefit was found when clopidogrel loading dose was administered 4-8 hours before PCI.

The CURRENT-OASIS 7 study, was a randomized, 2 x 2 factorial design trial evaluating a clopidogrel high-dose regimen (600 mg loading dose on day 1 followed by 150 mg once daily on days 2 to 7, followed by 75 mg once daily on days 8-30) compared with the standard-dose regimen (300 mg loading dose on day 1, followed by 75 mg once daily on days 2-30) and high-dose aspirin (300-325 mg daily) versus low-dose aspirin (75-100 mg daily) in patients with ST or non-ST-segment-elevation ACS managed with an early invasive strategy no later than 72 hours after randomization. The primary outcome was the composite of death from cardiovascular causes, myocardial (re)-infarction or stroke up to day 30. The primary safety outcome was major bleeding. The results of the CURRENT OASIS-7 presented at the European Society of Cardiology 2009 Congress (Barcelona, Spain) support doubling the loading and maintenance doses of clopidogrel in ACS patients undergoing planned PCI. This strategy significantly reduced stent thrombosis and cardiovascular events in the PCI cohort (17.232 patients), largely driven by reductions in myocardial infarction, with a significant increase in major or severe bleeding according to CURRENT definition. However, the trial failed to meet its primary end point in the overall cohort (25.087 patients) and the absolute effect in the PCI cohort was modest. In addition, there was no difference in the safety or efficacy of higher-dose aspirin when compared with lower-dose aspirin.

Safety and efficacy of clopidogrel daily maintenance dose higher than 75 mg remains uncertain. Angiolillo et al [77] showed that diabetic patients receiving 150 mg clopidogrel daily maintenance dose showed higher platelet inhibition than those receiving 75 mg; however, response to antiplatelet therapy remained highly variable and suboptimal clopidogrel response was still present in 60% of patients receiving 150 mg/day; in addition, this trial was not powered to evaluate clinical outcomes and bleeding events. Von Beckerath et al [78] have shown in stable patients undergoing successful PCI after administration of 600 mg clopidogrel loading dose more intense inhibition of platelet aggregation with 150 mg compared with 75 mg daily maintenance dose, but potential clinical benefits were not explored in this trial. Current guidelines do not recommend clopidogrel daily maintenance dose higher than 75 mg [32-34, 75, 76].

# Optimise Clopidogrel Response According to Platelet Function Tests

With regard to optimise clopidogrel response according to platelet function tests, Neubauer et al [79] had proposed in a observational study with stable patients, pre-treated with 600 mg clopidogrel loading dose followed by 75 mg daily maintenance dose undergoing elective PCI, an algorithm to reduce the incidence of clopidogrel resistance assessed by impedance aggregometry and evaluate therapeutic options: low responders received an additional 600 mg clopidogrel loading dose followed by 75 mg twice a day maintenance dose; in case of persistence of low response to clopidogrel high dose regimen, the antiplatelet therapy was changed to ticlopidine 250 mg twice daily. The incidence of low response to clopidogrel was reduced from 23.6% to 5.0%; nevertheless, this study lacks a clinical follow-up of patients to prove if optimised therapy translates into a reduction of cardiovascular events. Similarly, Bonello et al [80] have shown that in patients scheduled for elective PCI after 600 mg clopidogrel loading dose, adjusting the clopidogrel loading dose according to the results of platelet function assessed with the VASP assay is feasible, safe, and efficacious in reducing post-PCI MACE. In this trial, clopidogrel resistance was defined as a VASP-index >50% after 600 mg clopidogrel loading dose; thus, patients in the assay-guidance group were allowed up to three additional clopidogrel loading dose of 600 mg each, given successively as needed every 24 hours until the VASP-index dropped below 50%, prior PCI. Patients receiving standard clopidogrel loading dose compared to patients receiving VASP index-guided clopidogrel loading dose suffered higher rates of MACE at 30-day follow up (10% vs. 0%, p=0.007), without higher incidence of major or minor bleeding (5% vs. 4%, p=NS). However, due to the small sample size and the lower event rate registered (fewer than expected), these results should be taken into account cautiously before putting then into practice in a clinical basis.

Several PPR cut-off values have been proposed subsequent to platelet function assessed with the VerifyNow P2Y12 assay (Accumetrics Inc, San Diego, California): 175 PRU identified patients with NSTE-ACS undergoing early coronary angiography as being at higher risk for MACE at 1 year follow-up [30]; ≥240 PRU identified patients with ACS (STEMI and NSTEACS patients) who underwent PCI with a significantly higher risk of cardiovascular death and nonfatal myocardial infarction at 1-year follow-up [81]; ≥235 PRU identified patients (>90% with stable angina) following PCI with DES with significantly higher incidence of MACE at 6-months follow-up, including stent thrombosis [82]. The correct treatment, if any, of high PPR remains unknown pending the completion of currently ongoing clinical trials: the GRAVITAS (NCT00645918), the DANTE (NCT00774475), the ARCTIC (NCT00827411), and the TRIGGER-PCI (NCT00910299), which may reveal whether individualized antiplatelet treatment based on platelet function testing improves outcome. Until then, clinical practice should not be guided by (point-of-care) platelet function testing and current guidelines do not support this management. A position paper [83] of the Working Group on Thrombosis of the European Society of Cardiology do not support the routine or even the occasional determination and/or monitoring of platelet function while on therapy with antiplatelet drugs and subsequent therapeutic decisions.

# Chapter VI

# Emerging Therapies

The same studies that have established the safety and effectiveness of clopidogrel have also indicated the significant variable response associated with this treatment. In a way to improve the benefits of antiplatelet treatment, a new generation of P2Y12-ADP receptor antagonists has been developed. These new agents (Prasugrel, Cangrelor and Ticagrelor) are more potent, with a more rapid onset of action and less inter-individual variability. Table 3 summarizes current P2Y12-ADP receptor inhibitors.

**Table 3. P2Y$_{12}$-ADP Receptor Inhibitors**

|  | Clopidogrel | Prasugrel | Cangrelor | Tcagrelor |
|---|---|---|---|---|
| Group | Thienopyridine | Thienopyridine | ATP analogue | Cyclopentyl-triazolo-pyrimidine |
| Administration | Oral | Oral | Parenteral | Oral |
| Biodisponibility | Prodrug | Prodrug | Direct-acting | Direct-acting |
| Receptor Inhibition | Irreversible | Irreversible | Reversible | Reversible |
| Dose Frequency | Once daily | Once daily | Bolus and infusion | Twice daily |

# Prasugrel

Prasugrel is a third-generation thienopyridine that selective and irreversibly blocks the P2Y12-ADP receptor, with much more rapid and consistent inhibitory effects on platelet aggregation than clopidogrel. Prasugrel is a prodrug with rapid and almost complete absorption after oral ingestion of a loading dose. Its distinct chemical structure permits conversion to its active metabolite with less dependence on CYP enzymes than clopidogrel.

Prasugrel (60 mg loading dose followed by 10 mg daily maintenance dose), compared to clopidogrel (600 mg loading dose followed by 75 mg [84] or 150 mg [85] daily maintenance dose), provides faster onset, greater inhibition and less variability of P2Y12-ADP receptor-mediated platelet aggregation because of greater and more efficient generation of its active metabolite (in circulating blood within 15 minutes of dosing, which reaches maximal plasma concentration at 30 minutes). Other advantages of prasugrel over clopidogrel are that CYP genotype has no influence on its pharmacokinetics and pharmacodynamics and the much lower interindividual variability in the inhibition of P2Y12 dependent platelet responses leading to an extremely low prevalence of subjects who display resistance to prasugrel.

In the TRITON-TIMI 38 trial, patients with NSTE-ACS or STEMI undergoing PCI were randomly assigned to receive either prasugrel (60 mg loading dose followed by 10 mg daily maintenance dose) or clopidogrel (300 mg loading dose followed by 75 mg daily maintenance dose). A significant decrease in the combined primary end point (death from cardiovascular cause, nonfatal myocardial infarction, or stroke) was found with prasugrel as compared with clopidogrel, but a significant excess of TIMI major bleeding, life-threatening bleeding and fatal bleeding was shown in patients assigned to prasugrel, so that, for each death from cardiovascular causes prevented by the use of prasugrel compared with clopidogrel, approximately one additional episode of fatal bleeding was caused by prasugrel, leading to similar net clinical benefit with no significant differences in death from any cause [86]. In the TRITON-TIMI 38, the loading dose of clopidogrel was 300 mg (the FDA-approved regimen), while in the PRINCIPLE-TIMI 44 [85], prasugrel was compared to 600 mg loading dose of clopidogrel, a regimen increasingly used in patients undergoing PCI. Subsequent analysis has shown that the net clinical benefit with prasugrel was greater for patients with diabetes than for patients without diabetes, including a gradient from no DM to DM without insulin therapy to DM with insulin therapy [87].

In summary, in the TRITON-TIMI 38 studies the main topics to point out are:

1. prasugrel significantly reduces the risks of recurrent myocardial infarction (spontaneous and procedural) and stent thrombosis as compared with clopidogrel.
2. these benefits are particularly sizable among patients with diabetes or ST-segment elevation.
3. the finding of an approximately 50% reduction in the rate of stent thrombosis (for both drug-eluting and bare-metal stents) supports the use of prasugrel after PCI.
4. there is an excess of major bleeding events in prasugrel treated patients, leading to similar net clinical benefit.

Concerning the increase in bleeding events associated to prasugrel therapy, three subgroups appeared to be particularly prone to serious bleeding: the elderly (75 years of age or older), the underweight (weigh less than 60 kg), and patients with a previous stroke or transient ischemic attack. Therefore, it would be the best to avoid prasugrel therapy in such patients. Reduce loading and maintenance dose is an alternative approach, but there is no direct evidence that efficacy would be maintained. However, it should be noticed that older patients in two subgroups at particularly high thrombotic risk (patients with diabetes and patients with a prior myocardial infarction) appeared to benefit substantially from prasugrel. Therefore, choosing a therapy requires balancing the reduction in the risk of thrombotic events against the bleeding risk.

A small number of patients underwent CABG. Among these patients, the rate of major bleeding in the prasugrel group was more than four times that in the clopidogrel group (13.4% vs. 3.2%). Then, early prasugrel treatment without delineation of the coronary anatomy by cardiac catheterization should not be routine in patients with unstable angina/myocardial infarction without ST-segment elevation.

Finally, on July 10, 2009, after an 18-month review, the Food and Drug Administration (FDA) approved the prasugrel (60 mg loading dose followed by 10 mg daily maintenance dose) for use in patients with unstable angina or myocardial infarction who undergo PCI. The clinical efficacy of prasugrel in patients with NSTE-ACS following medical treatment will be tested in the TRILOGY-SCA trial (Targeted Platelet Inhibition to Clarify the Optimal Strategy to Medically Manage Acute Coronary Syndromes) (NCT00699998).

# Ticagrelor

Ticagrelor, previously known as AZD6140, belongs to the new chemical class cyclopentyl-triazolo-pyrimidines. Ticagrelor is an oral direct-acting P2Y12 inhibitor that changes the conformation of the P2Y12 receptor leading to a reversible inhibition of the receptor without the need for any metabolic activation. The plasma half-life is 6-13 hours and therefore the treatment is given twice daily. Ticagrelor provides faster, greater and more consistent P2Y12 inhibition than clopidogrel [88].

The safety, tolerability, and efficacy of ticagrelor plus aspirin in comparison with clopidogrel plus aspirin were initially evaluated in patients with NSTE-ACS in the DISPERSE-2 study [89] (a randomized, double-blind, double-dummy trial). No difference in major bleeding but an increase in minor bleeding occurred with ticagrelor 90 mg twice daily compared to clopidogrel 75 mg once daily.

In the PLATO trial [90] (a phase III randomized, double-blind, parallel group efficacy and safety study enrolling 18,624 patients), ticagrelor (180-mg loading dose, 90 mg twice daily thereafter) was compared to clopidogrel (300-to-600-mg loading dose, 75 mg daily thereafter) for the prevention of cardiovascular events in patients admitted to the hospital with ACS, with or without ST-segment elevation. After 12 months of follow-up, the primary end point (a composite of vascular death, myocardial infarction, or stroke) occurred in 9.8% of patients receiving ticagrelor compared with 11.7% of patients receiving clopidogrel. There was a higher incidence of TIMI major non-CABG related bleeding in patients who received ticagrelor (2.8%) compared with those treated with clopidogrel (2.2%; P=0.03). However, the incidence of TIMI major CABG related bleeding was similar in the 2 groups. Because of the rather high incidence of CABG-related bleeding in both groups (446 of 931 [47.9%] in ticagrelor-treated patients versus 476 of 968 [49.2%] in clopidogrel-treated patients), the incidence of total bleeding was not significantly different. Therefore, consistent with TRITON-TIMI 38, the PLATO trial showed that a more consistent, adequate inhibition of P2Y12-dependent platelet function is associated with greater antithrombotic efficacy and increased risk of non CABG-related major bleeding. Treatment with ticagrelor was more advantageous than treatment with clopidogrel in patients undergoing CABG; in fact, the 2 treatments were associated with similar incidences of CABG-related bleeding despite the fact that ticagrelor had been withheld for only 24 to 72 hours before surgery compared with clopidogrel, which had been withheld for 5 days. The results of the PLATO-CABG analysis have been reported in the American College of Cardiology 2010 Scientific Sessions (Atlanta, Georgia, USA). This analysis was intended to evaluate the efficacy and safety of ticagrelor in comparison with clopidogrel after CABG, in patients with last intake of study drug within seven days of surgery. There was no difference in the composite primary end point between the two study arms or in the rates of MI or stroke. Cardiovascular death was reduced by 50% in the ticagrelor arm, despite the absence of any difference in bleeding between the clopidogrel and ticagrelor arms.

Like the DISPERSE and DISPERSE-2 trials, the PLATO trial showed an increased incidence of dyspnea in ticagrelor-treated patients (13.8% versus 7.8%; P=0.001), which required discontinuation of the drug in 0.9% of patients (0.1% in the clopidogrel arm). There was a higher incidence of ventricular pauses of greater than or equal to 3 seconds in the first week in the ticagrelor group compared to clopidogrel group, without significant differences in the incidence of syncope or pacemaker implantation. The levels of creatinine and uric acid increased slightly more with ticagrelor than with clopidogrel during the treatment period.

The results of the PLATO trial were confirmed in the subgroup of patients following an invasive management. The PLATO INVASIVE substudy [91] showed that ACS patients undergoing an early invasive strategy (13408 patients -

72% of the study population-) have significantly lower rates of cardiovascular death, ischemic events and stent thrombosis at 1 year follow-up with ticagrelor as compared with clopidogrel. This study also clarifies that the overall benefits of ticagrelor versus clopidogrel were identical regardless of the loading dose of clopidogrel. As previously described in the overall study population of the PLATO trial, the rate of major or minor bleeding events non-CABG-related were significantly higher in the ticagrelor group (8.9% in ticagrelor-treated patients versus 7.1% in clopidogrel-treated patients; P=0.0004), with no significant difference in the rates of total major bleeding o severe bleeding according to the GUSTO classification.

In the same way, ticagrelor was superior to clopidogrel in a subset of 8430 STEMI patients undergoing planned PCI. The results of this predefined subanalysis of PLATO were reported during a late-breaking clinical-trial session at the American Heart Association 2009 Scientific Sessions (Orland, Florida, USA) [92]. Definite stent thrombosis, myocardial infarction and all-cause mortality was significantly lower among STEMI patients taking ticagrelor compared with those receiving clopidogrel, with no significant difference in the rates of total major bleeding.

In addition, in patients with stable coronary artery disease who are already taking aspirin therapy [93], ticagrelor compared with clopidogrel, achieves more rapid and greater platelet inhibition, continued during the maintenance phase, and the offset of action is faster with ticagrelor therapy than with clopidogrel. These pharmacodynamic effects may explain why ticagrelor treatment was associated with a lower occurrence of the primary end point (myocardial infarction, stroke, or cardiovascular death), similar coronary artery bypass graft-related bleeding, and no overall difference in major bleeding compared with clopidogrel therapy in the PLATO trial.

The RESPOND study [94] enrolled 98 patients with stable coronary artery disease on aspirin therapy and has shown that ticagrelor therapy overcomes non-responsiveness to clopidogrel and high platelet reactivity during clopidogrel therapy. In addition, the antiplatelet effect of ticagrelor was essentially uniform and high in both clopidogrel responders and non-responders; there was an extremely low prevalence of high platelet reactivity associated with ticagrelor therapy and platelet inhibition was enhanced by switching to ticagrelor therapy in both patients responsive and non-responsive to clopidogrel. These data suggest that ticagrelor may be an important therapeutic alternative in patients who have experienced thrombotic events during clopidogrel therapy. The authors state that all of these findings support the particular utility of ticagrelor in clinical settings associated with high platelet reactivity, such as ACS, PCI and stent thrombosis. However, this study only enrolled patients with stable coronary artery disease, was unpowered to investigate safety end points and these results were not correlated with thrombotic events at follow-up.

In summary, ticagrelor compared to clopidogrel, has a more rapid onset, pronounced and consistent platelet inhibition, with faster offset after cessation. The adverse effects of ticagrelor may require evaluation in a much larger number of patients to establish the overall impact before drawing definitive conclusions. Given the potential adverse effects described, the use of ticagrelor should be done with caution in patients with an excessively high risk of bleeding, and should be avoided in case of chronic obstructive pulmonary disease, hyperuricemia, moderate or severe renal failure, bradyarrhythmias unprotected by pacemakers or a history of syncope.

# Cangrelor

Cangrelor, a nonthienopyridine ATP analogue, is a potent direct-acting, selective, and specific inhibitor of the ADP receptor P2Y12. Cangrelor does not require conversion to an active metabolite, therefore, is immediately active after intravenous infusion with a plasma half-life of 3 to 6 minutes, and is metabolized through dephosphorylation pathways. Platelet function normalizes within 30 to 60 minutes after discontinuation.

A large, 2-part phase II study [95] assessed the safety and pharmacodynamics of cangrelor in patients undergoing PCI. The first part of the study enrolled 200 patients undergoing PCI who were randomized to an 18- to 24-hours intravenous infusion of placebo or to 1, 2, or 4 μg/Kg-min cangrelor in addition to aspirin and heparin before the procedure. In the second part of the study, 199 patients were randomized to receive either cangrelor (4 μg/Kg-min) or the anti-glycoprotein IIb/IIIa inhibitor abciximab before the procedure. The incidence of combined major and minor bleeding was not significantly higher in cangrelor-treated patients compared with placebo- or abciximab-treated patients. Mean inhibition of platelet aggregation in response to 3 μmol/L ADP was complete in both the group of patients treated with cangrelor 4 μg/Kg-min and the group treated with abciximab. However, after termination of drug infusion, platelet aggregation returned to baseline values much faster in the cangrelor-treated group than in the abciximab-treated group. These data suggest that cangrelor may be useful during the periprocedural period in patients undergoing PCI. However, for long-term prevention, these patients should be treated with orally available agents.

Two large, phase 3, randomized clinical trials [96, 97] comparing cangrelor with clopidogrel have been made recently in order to establish the role of cangrelor in patients with acute coronary syndrome undergoing elective PCI. The major difference between the two trials was the timing of the administration of the study drugs. In the CHAMPION PCI [97] (with a double-blind, double-dummy design), cangrelor administered 30 minutes before PCI (30 µg /kg bolus followed by 4µg/Kg/min infusion and continued for 2 hours after PCI) was compared to clopidogrel administered 30 minutes before PCI (600 mg loading dose). Patients in the cangrelor group received received 600 mg clopidogrel loading after the end of the cangrelor infusion. In the CHAMPION PLATFORM [96] (double-blind, placebo controlled sudy), cangrelor was started at the beginning of PCI (30 µg /kg bolus followed by 4µg/Kg/min infusion with a minumum duration time of 2 hours, and a maximum duration time of 4 hours), whereas clopidogrel (600 mg loading dose) was not administered before the end of PCI. Patients in the cangrelor group received received 600 mg of clopidogrel after the end of the cangrelor infusion.

In the two CHAMPION trials, an interim analysis concluded that cangrelor would not show superiority for the composite primary end point and enrollment was stopped. So that, cangrelor was not superior to an oral loading dose of 600 mg of clopidogrel reducing the composite end point of death from any cause, myocardial infarction, or ischemia-driven revascularization at 48 hours. However, in the CHAMPION PLATFORM trial, in the cangrelor group, as compared with the placebo group, two prespecified secondary end points were significantly reduced at 48 hours: the rate of stent thrombosis, from 0.6% to 0.2% (odds ratio, 0.31; 95% CI, 0.11 to 0.85; $P = 0.02$), and the rate of death from any cause, from 0.7% to 0.2% (odds ratio, 0.33; 95% CI, 0.13 to 0.83; $P = 0.02$).

The most important lesson from the two CHAMPION trials is that in patients with ACS in whom the administration of an P2Y12-ADP receptor antagonist was deferred until diagnostic angiography had established the indication for PCI, intravenous cangrelor did not provide additional advantages to those achieved with 600 mg of clopidogrel. However, cangrelor is a potent intravenous P2Y12-ADP receptor inhibitor with a rapid onset and offset of action. These valuable qualities certainly warrant further studies aimed at identifying more suitable clinical scenarios for cangrelor and more appropriate approaches to its use.

# References

[1]     Ibanez B, Vilahur G, Badimon JJ. Plaque progression and regression in atherothrombosis. *J Thromb Haemost.* 2007;5 Suppl 1:292-299.

[2]     Fuster V, Fayad ZA, Moreno PR, Poon M, Corti R, Badimon JJ. Atherothrombosis and high-risk plaque: Part II: approaches by noninvasive computed tomographic/magnetic resonance imaging. *J Am Coll Cardiol.* 2005;46(7):1209-1218.

[3]     Cattaneo M. Resistance to antiplatelet drugs: molecular mechanisms and laboratory detection. *J Thromb Haemost.* 2007;5 Suppl 1:230-237.

[4]     Gachet C. P2 receptors, platelet function and pharmacological implications. *Thromb Haemost.* 2008;99(3):466-472.

[5]     Ibanez BV, G. Badimon, J. Pharmacology of thienopyridines: rationale for dual pathway inhibition. *European Heart Journal* 2006;Suppl 8:G3-G9.

[6]     Mehta SR, Yusuf S, Peters RJ, Bertrand ME, Lewis BS, Natarajan MK, Malmberg K, Rupprecht H, Zhao F, Chrolavicius S, Copland I, Fox KA. Effects of pretreatment with clopidogrel and aspirin followed by long-term therapy in patients undergoing percutaneous coronary intervention: the PCI-CURE study. *Lancet.* 2001;358(9281):527-533.

[7]     Sabatine MS, Cannon CP, Gibson CM, Lopez-Sendon JL, Montalescot G, Theroux P, Lewis BS, Murphy SA, McCabe CH, Braunwald E. Effect of clopidogrel pretreatment before percutaneous coronary intervention in patients with ST-elevation myocardial infarction treated with fibrinolytics: the PCI-CLARITY study. *JAMA.* 2005;294(10):1224-1232.

[8]     Steinhubl SR, Berger PB, Mann JT, 3rd, Fry ET, DeLago A, Wilmer C, Topol EJ. Early and sustained dual oral antiplatelet therapy following percutaneous coronary intervention: a randomized controlled trial. *JAMA.* 2002;288(19):2411-2420.

[9]   Yusuf S, Zhao F, Mehta SR, Chrolavicius S, Tognoni G, Fox KK. Effects of clopidogrel in addition to aspirin in patients with acute coronary syndromes without ST-segment elevation. *N Engl J Med.* 2001;345(7):494-502.

[10]  Chen ZM, Jiang LX, Chen YP, Xie JX, Pan HC, Peto R, Collins R, Liu LS. Addition of clopidogrel to aspirin in 45,852 patients with acute myocardial infarction: randomised placebo-controlled trial. *Lancet.* 2005;366(9497):1607-1621.

[11]  Sabatine MS, Cannon CP, Gibson CM, Lopez-Sendon JL, Montalescot G, Theroux P, Claeys MJ, Cools F, Hill KA, Skene AM, McCabe CH, Braunwald E. Addition of clopidogrel to aspirin and fibrinolytic therapy for myocardial infarction with ST-segment elevation. *N Engl J Med.* 2005;352(12):1179-1189.

[12]  Zeymer U, Gitt A, Junger C, Bauer T, Heer T, Koeth O, Mark B, Zahn R, Senges J, Gottwik M. Clopidogrel in addition to aspirin reduces in-hospital major cardiac and cerebrovascular events in unselected patients with acute ST segment elevation myocardial. *Thromb Haemost.* 2008;99(1):155-160.

[13]  Bhatt DL, Fox KA, Hacke W, Berger PB, Black HR, Boden WE, Cacoub P, Cohen EA, Creager MA, Easton JD, Flather MD, Haffner SM, Hamm CW, Hankey GJ, Johnston SC, Mak KH, Mas JL, Montalescot G, Pearson TA, Steg PG, Steinhubl SR, Weber MA, Brennan DM, Fabry-Ribaudo L, Booth J, Topol EJ. Clopidogrel and aspirin versus aspirin alone for the prevention of atherothrombotic events. *N Engl J Med.* 2006;354(16):1706-1717.

[14]  Lev EI, Patel RT, Maresh KJ, Guthikonda S, Granada J, DeLao T, Bray PF, Kleiman NS. Aspirin and clopidogrel drug response in patients undergoing percutaneous coronary intervention: the role of dual drug resistance. *J Am Coll Cardiol.* 2006;47(1):27-33.

[15]  Gurbel PA, Bliden KP, Hayes KM, Yoho JA, Herzog WR, Tantry US. The relation of dosing to clopidogrel responsiveness and the incidence of high post-treatment platelet aggregation in patients undergoing coronary stenting. *J Am Coll Cardiol.* 2005;45(9):1392-1396.

[16]  Matetzky S, Shenkman B, Guetta V, Shechter M, Bienart R, Goldenberg I, Novikov I, Pres H, Savion N, Varon D, Hod H. Clopidogrel resistance is associated with increased risk of recurrent atherothrombotic events in patients with acute myocardial infarction. *Circulation.* 2004;109(25):3171-3175.

[17]  Muller I, Besta F, Schulz C, Massberg S, Schonig A, Gawaz M. Prevalence of clopidogrel non-responders among patients with stable angina pectoris scheduled for elective coronary stent placement. *Thromb Haemost.* 2003;89(5):783-787.

[18] Jaremo P, Lindahl TL, Fransson SG, Richter A. Individual variations of platelet inhibition after loading doses of clopidogrel. *J Intern Med.* 2002;252(3):233-238.

[19] Mobley JE, Bresee SJ, Wortham DC, Craft RM, Snider CC, Carroll RC. Frequency of nonresponse antiplatelet activity of clopidogrel during pretreatment for cardiac catheterization. *Am J Cardiol.* 2004;93(4):456-458.

[20] Lepantalo A, Virtanen KS, Heikkila J, Wartiovaara U, Lassila R. Limited early antiplatelet effect of 300 mg clopidogrel in patients with aspirin therapy undergoing percutaneous coronary interventions. *Eur Heart J.* 2004;25(6):476-483.

[21] Angiolillo DJ, Fernandez-Ortiz A, Bernardo E, Ramirez C, Barrera-Ramirez C, Sabate M, Hernandez R, Moreno R, Escaned J, Alfonso F, Banuelos C, Costa MA, Bass TA, Macaya C. Identification of low responders to a 300-mg clopidogrel loading dose in patients undergoing coronary stenting. *Thromb Res.* 2005;115(1-2):101-108.

[22] Dziewierz A, Dudek D, Heba G, Rakowski T, Mielecki W, Dubiel JS. Inter-individual variability in response to clopidogrel in patients with coronary artery disease. *Kardiol Pol.* 2005;62(2):108-117; discussion 118.

[23] Serebruany VL, Steinhubl SR, Berger PB, Malinin AI, Bhatt DL, Topol EJ. Variability in platelet responsiveness to clopidogrel among 544 individuals. *J Am Coll Cardiol.* 2005;45(2):246-251.

[24] Hochholzer W, Trenk D, Bestehorn HP, Fischer B, Valina CM, Ferenc M, Gick M, Caputo A, Buttner HJ, Neumann FJ. Impact of the degree of peri-interventional platelet inhibition after loading with clopidogrel on early clinical outcome of elective coronary stent placement. *J Am Coll Cardiol.* 2006;48(9):1742-1750.

[25] Cuisset T, Frere C, Quilici J, Morange PE, Nait-Saidi L, Carvajal J, Lehmann A, Lambert M, Bonnet JL, Alessi MC. Benefit of a 600-mg loading dose of clopidogrel on platelet reactivity and clinical outcomes in patients with non-ST-segment elevation acute coronary syndrome undergoing coronary stenting. *J Am Coll Cardiol.* 2006;48(7):1339-1345.

[26] Campo G, Valgimigli M, Gemmati D, Percoco G, Tognazzo S, Cicchitelli G, Catozzi L, Malagutti P, Anselmi M, Vassanelli C, Scapoli G, Ferrari R. Value of platelet reactivity in predicting response to treatment and clinical outcome in patients undergoing primary coronary intervention: insights into the STRATEGY Study. *J Am Coll Cardiol.* 2006;48(11):2178-2185.

[27] Gurbel PA, Bliden KP, Guyer K, Cho PW, Zaman KA, Kreutz RP, Bassi AK, Tantry US. Platelet reactivity in patients and recurrent events post-stenting: results of the PREPARE POST-STENTING Study. *J Am Coll Cardiol.* 2005;46(10):1820-1826.

[28] Samara WM, Bliden KP, Tantry US, Gurbel PA. The difference between clopidogrel responsiveness and posttreatment platelet reactivity. *Thromb Res.* 2005;115(1-2):89-94.

[29] Bliden KP, DiChiara J, Tantry US, Bassi AK, Chaganti SK, Gurbel PA. Increased risk in patients with high platelet aggregation receiving chronic clopidogrel therapy undergoing percutaneous coronary intervention: is the current antiplatelet therapy adequate? *J Am Coll Cardiol.* 2007;49(6):657-666.

[30] de Miguel Castro A, Cuellas Ramon C, Diego Nieto A, Samaniego Lampon B, Alonso Rodriguez D, Fernandez Vazquez F, Alonso Orcajo N, Carbonell de Blas R, Pascual Vicente C, Perez de Prado A. Post-treatment platelet reactivity predicts long-term adverse events better than the response to clopidogrel in patients with non-ST-segment elevation acute coronary syndrome. *Rev Esp Cardiol.* 2009;62(2):126-135.

[31] Hovens MM, Snoep JD, Eikenboom JC, van der Bom JG, Mertens BJ, Huisman MV. Prevalence of persistent platelet reactivity despite use of aspirin: a systematic review. *Am Heart J.* 2007;153(2):175-181.

[32] King SB, 3rd, Smith SC, Jr., Hirshfeld JW, Jr., Jacobs AK, Morrison DA, Williams DO, Feldman TE, Kern MJ, O'Neill WW, Schaff HV, Whitlow PL, Adams CD, Anderson JL, Buller CE, Creager MA, Ettinger SM, Halperin JL, Hunt SA, Krumholz HM, Kushner FG, Lytle BW, Nishimura R, Page RL, Riegel B, Tarkington LG, Yancy CW. 2007 focused update of the ACC/AHA/SCAI 2005 guideline update for percutaneous coronary intervention: a report of the American College of Cardiology/American Heart Association Task Force on Practice guidelines. *J Am Coll Cardiol.* 2008;51(2):172-209.

[33] Anderson JL, Adams CD, Antman EM, Bridges CR, Califf RM, Casey DE, Jr., Chavey WE, 2nd, Fesmire FM, Hochman JS, Levin TN, Lincoff AM, Peterson ED, Theroux P, Wenger NK, Wright RS, Smith SC, Jr., Jacobs AK, Halperin JL, Hunt SA, Krumholz HM, Kushner FG, Lytle BW, Nishimura R, Ornato JP, Page RL, Riegel B. ACC/AHA 2007 guidelines for the management of patients with unstable angina/non-ST-Elevation myocardial infarction: a report of the American College of Cardiology/American Heart Association Task Force on Practice Guidelines (Writing Committee to Revise the 2002 Guidelines for the Management of Patients With Unstable Angina/Non-ST-Elevation Myocardial Infarction) developed in collaboration with the American College of Emergency Physicians, the Society for Cardiovascular Angiography and Interventions, and the Society of Thoracic Surgeons endorsed by the American Association of Cardiovascular and Pulmonary Rehabilitation and the

Society for Academic Emergency Medicine. *J Am Coll Cardiol.* 2007;50(7):e1-e157.

[34] Bassand JP, Hamm CW, Ardissino D, Boersma E, Budaj A, Fernandez-Aviles F, Fox KA, Hasdai D, Ohman EM, Wallentin L, Wijns W. Guidelines for the diagnosis and treatment of non-ST-segment elevation acute coronary syndromes. *Eur Heart J.* 2007;28(13):1598-1660.

[35] Simoons ML. Effect of glycoprotein IIb/IIIa receptor blocker abciximab on outcome in patients with acute coronary syndromes without early coronary revascularisation: the GUSTO IV-ACS randomised trial. *Lancet.* 2001;357(9272):1915-1924.

[36] Topol EJ. Reperfusion therapy for acute myocardial infarction with fibrinolytic therapy or combination reduced fibrinolytic therapy and platelet glycoprotein IIb/IIIa inhibition: the GUSTO V randomised trial. *Lancet.* 2001;357(9272):1905-1914.

[37] Brandt JT, Close SL, Iturria SJ, Payne CD, Farid NA, Ernest CS, 2nd, Lachno DR, Salazar D, Winters KJ. Common polymorphisms of CYP2C19 and CYP2C9 affect the pharmacokinetic and pharmacodynamic response to clopidogrel but not prasugrel. *J Thromb Haemost.* 2007;5(12):2429-2436.

[38] Trenk D, Hochholzer W, Fromm MF, Chialda LE, Pahl A, Valina CM, Stratz C, Schmiebusch P, Bestehorn HP, Buttner HJ, Neumann FJ. Cytochrome P450 2C19 681G>A polymorphism and high on-clopidogrel platelet reactivity associated with adverse 1-year clinical outcome of elective percutaneous coronary intervention with drug-eluting or bare-metal stents. *J Am Coll Cardiol.* 2008;51(20):1925-1934.

[39] Mega JL, Close SL, Wiviott SD, Shen L, Hockett RD, Brandt JT, Walker JR, Antman EM, Macias W, Braunwald E, Sabatine MS. Cytochrome p-450 polymorphisms and response to clopidogrel. *N Engl J Med.* 2009;360(4):354-362.

[40] Lau WC, Waskell LA, Watkins PB, Neer CJ, Horowitz K, Hopp AS, Tait AR, Carville DG, Guyer KE, Bates ER. Atorvastatin reduces the ability of clopidogrel to inhibit platelet aggregation: a new drug-drug interaction. *Circulation.* 2003;107(1):32-37.

[41] Neubauer H, Gunesdogan B, Hanefeld C, Spiecker M, Mugge A. Lipophilic statins interfere with the inhibitory effects of clopidogrel on platelet function--a flow cytometry study. *Eur Heart J.* 2003;24(19):1744-1749.

[42] Mitsios JV, Papathanasiou AI, Rodis FI, Elisaf M, Goudevenos JA, Tselepis AD. Atorvastatin does not affect the antiplatelet potency of clopidogrel when it is administered concomitantly for 5 weeks in patients with acute coronary syndromes. *Circulation.* 2004;109(11):1335-1338.

[43] Gorchakova O, von Beckerath N, Gawaz M, Mocz A, Joost A, Schomig A, Kastrati A. Antiplatelet effects of a 600 mg loading dose of clopidogrel are

not attenuated in patients receiving atorvastatin or simvastatin for at least 4 weeks prior to coronary artery stenting. *Eur Heart J.* 2004;25(21):1898-1902.

[44]    Bhatt DL, Scheiman J, Abraham NS, Antman EM, Chan FK, Furberg CD, Johnson DA, Mahaffey KW, Quigley EM, Harrington RA, Bates ER, Bridges CR, Eisenberg MJ, Ferrari VA, Hlatky MA, Kaul S, Lindner JR, Moliterno DJ, Mukherjee D, Schofield RS, Rosenson RS, Stein JH, Weitz HH, Wesley DJ. ACCF/ACG/AHA 2008 expert consensus document on reducing the gastrointestinal risks of antiplatelet therapy and NSAID use. *Am J Gastroenterol.* 2008;103(11):2890-2907.

[45]    Gilard M, Arnaud B, Cornily JC, Le Gal G, Lacut K, Le Calvez G, Mansourati J, Mottier D, Abgrall JF, Boschat J. Influence of omeprazole on the antiplatelet action of clopidogrel associated with aspirin: the randomized, double-blind OCLA (Omeprazole CLopidogrel Aspirin) study. *J Am Coll Cardiol.* 2008;51(3):256-260.

[46]    Sibbing D, Morath T, Stegherr J, Braun S, Vogt W, Hadamitzky M, Schomig A, Kastrati A, von Beckerath N. Impact of proton pump inhibitors on the antiplatelet effects of clopidogrel. *Thromb Haemost.* 2009;101(4):714-719.

[47]    Cuisset T, Frere C, Quilici J, Poyet R, Gaborit B, Bali L, Brissy O, Morange PE, Alessi MC, Bonnet JL. Comparison of omeprazole and pantoprazole influence on a high 150-mg clopidogrel maintenance dose the PACA (Proton Pump Inhibitors And Clopidogrel Association) prospective randomized study. *J Am Coll Cardiol.* 2009;54(13):1149-1153.

[48]    Gaglia MA, Jr., Torguson R, Hanna N, Gonzalez MA, Collins SD, Syed AI, Ben-Dor I, Maluenda G, Delhaye C, Wakabayashi K, Xue Z, Suddath WO, Kent KM, Satler LF, Pichard AD, Waksman R. Relation of proton pump inhibitor use after percutaneous coronary intervention with drug-eluting stents to outcomes. *Am J Cardiol.*105(6):833-838.

[49]    Ho PM, Maddox TM, Wang L, Fihn SD, Jesse RL, Peterson ED, Rumsfeld JS. Risk of adverse outcomes associated with concomitant use of clopidogrel and proton pump inhibitors following acute coronary syndrome. *JAMA.* 2009;301(9):937-944.

[50]    Siller-Matula JM, Lang I, Christ G, Jilma B. Calcium-channel blockers reduce the antiplatelet effect of clopidogrel. *J Am Coll Cardiol.* 2008;52(19):1557-1563.

[51]    Gremmel T, Steiner S, Seidinger D, Koppensteiner R, Panzer S, Kopp CW. Calcium-channel blockers decrease clopidogrel-mediated platelet inhibition. *Heart.*96(3):186-189.

[52]    Michelson AD, Frelinger AL, 3rd, Furman MI. Current options in platelet function testing. *Am J Cardiol.* 2006;98(10A):4N-10N.

[53] Geisler T, Langer H, Wydymus M, Gohring K, Zurn C, Bigalke B, Stellos K, May AE, Gawaz M. Low response to clopidogrel is associated with cardiovascular outcome after coronary stent implantation. *Eur Heart J.* 2006;27(20):2420-2425.

[54] Breet NJ, van Werkum JW, Bouman HJ, Kelder JC, Ruven HJ, Bal ET, Deneer VH, Harmsze AM, van der Heyden JA, Rensing BJ, Suttorp MJ, Hackeng CM, ten Berg JM. Comparison of platelet function tests in predicting clinical outcome in patients undergoing coronary stent implantation. *JAMA.*303(8):754-762.

[55] Cuisset T, Frere C, Quilici J, Morange PE, Nait-Saidi L, Mielot C, Bali L, Lambert M, Alessi MC, Bonnet JL. High post-treatment platelet reactivity is associated with a high incidence of myonecrosis after stenting for non-ST elevation acute coronary syndromes. *Thromb Haemost.* 2007;97(2):282-287.

[56] Perez de Prado A, Cuellas C, Diego A, de Miguel A, Samaniego B, Alonso-Orcajo N, Carbonell R, Pascual C, Fernandez-Vazquez F, Calabozo RG. Influence of platelet reactivity and response to clopidogrel on myocardial damage following percutaneous coronary intervention in patients with non-ST-segment elevation acute coronary syndrome. *Thromb Res.* 2009;124(6):678-682.

[57] Marcucci R, Paniccia R, Antonucci E, Poli S, Gori AM, Valente S, Giglioli C, Lazzeri C, Prisco D, Abbate R, Gensini GF. Residual platelet reactivity is an independent predictor of myocardial injury in acute myocardial infarction patients on antiaggregant therapy. *Thromb Haemost.* 2007;98(4):844-851.

[58] Gurbel PA, Bliden KP, Samara W, Yoho JA, Hayes K, Fissha MZ, Tantry US. Clopidogrel effect on platelet reactivity in patients with stent thrombosis: results of the CREST Study. *J Am Coll Cardiol.* 2005;46(10):1827-1832.

[59] Stone GW, Moses JW, Ellis SG, Schofer J, Dawkins KD, Morice MC, Colombo A, Schampaert E, Grube E, Kirtane AJ, Cutlip DE, Fahy M, Pocock SJ, Mehran R, Leon MB. Safety and efficacy of sirolimus- and paclitaxel-eluting coronary stents. *N Engl J Med.* 2007;356(10):998-1008.

[60] Lagerqvist B, James SK, Stenestrand U, Lindback J, Nilsson T, Wallentin L. Long-term outcomes with drug-eluting stents versus bare-metal stents in Sweden. *N Engl J Med.* 2007;356(10):1009-1019.

[61] Iakovou I, Schmidt T, Bonizzoni E, Ge L, Sangiorgi GM, Stankovic G, Airoldi F, Chieffo A, Montorfano M, Carlino M, Michev I, Corvaja N, Briguori C, Gerckens U, Grube E, Colombo A. Incidence, predictors, and outcome of thrombosis after successful implantation of drug-eluting stents. *JAMA.* 2005;293(17):2126-2130.

[62] van Werkum JW, Heestermans AA, Zomer AC, Kelder JC, Suttorp MJ, Rensing BJ, Koolen JJ, Brueren BR, Dambrink JH, Hautvast RW, Verheugt

FW, ten Berg JM. Predictors of coronary stent thrombosis: the Dutch Stent Thrombosis Registry. *J Am Coll Cardiol.* 2009;53(16):1399-1409.

[63] Buonamici P, Marcucci R, Migliorini A, Gensini GF, Santini A, Paniccia R, Moschi G, Gori AM, Abbate R, Antoniucci D. Impact of platelet reactivity after clopidogrel administration on drug-eluting stent thrombosis. *J Am Coll Cardiol.* 2007;49(24):2312-2317.

[64] Sibbing D, Braun S, Morath T, Mehilli J, Vogt W, Schomig A, Kastrati A, von Beckerath N. Platelet reactivity after clopidogrel treatment assessed with point-of-care analysis and early drug-eluting stent thrombosis. *J Am Coll Cardiol.* 2009;53(10):849-856.

[65] Gori AM, Marcucci R, Migliorini A, Valenti R, Moschi G, Paniccia R, Buonamici P, Gensini GF, Vergara R, Abbate R, Antoniucci D. Incidence and clinical impact of dual nonresponsiveness to aspirin and clopidogrel in patients with drug-eluting stents. *J Am Coll Cardiol.* 2008;52(9):734-739.

[66] Geisler T, Zurn C, Simonenko R, Rapin M, Kraibooj H, Kilias A, Bigalke B, Stellos K, Schwab M, May AE, Herdeg C, Gawaz M. Early but not late stent thrombosis is influenced by residual platelet aggregation in patients undergoing coronary interventions. *Eur Heart J.*31(1):59-66.

[67] Sibbing D, Morath T, Braun S, Stegherr J, Mehilli J, Vogt W, Schomig A, Kastrati A, von Beckerath N. Clopidogrel response status assessed with Multiplate point-of-care analysis and the incidence and timing of stent thrombosis over six months following coronary stenting. *Thromb Haemost.*103(1):151-159.

[68] Grines CL, Bonow RO, Casey DE, Jr., Gardner TJ, Lockhart PB, Moliterno DJ, O'Gara P, Whitlow P. Prevention of premature discontinuation of dual antiplatelet therapy in patients with coronary artery stents: a science advisory from the American Heart Association, American College of Cardiology, Society for Cardiovascular Angiography and Interventions, American College of Surgeons, and American Dental Association, with representation from the American College of Physicians. *Circulation.* 2007;115(6):813-818.

[69] Park SJ, Park DW, Kim YH, Kang SJ, Lee SW, Lee CW, Han KH, Park SW, Yun SC, Lee SG, Rha SW, Seong IW, Jeong MH, Hur SH, Lee NH, Yoon J, Yang JY, Lee BK, Choi YJ, Chung WS, Lim DS, Cheong SS, Kim KS, Chae JK, Nah DY, Jeon DS, Seung KB, Jang JS, Park HS, Lee K. Duration of Dual Antiplatelet Therapy after Implantation of Drug-Eluting Stents. *N Engl J Med.*

[70] Muller I, Seyfarth M, Rudiger S, Wolf B, Pogatsa-Murray G, Schomig A, Gawaz M. Effect of a high loading dose of clopidogrel on platelet function in patients undergoing coronary stent placement. *Heart.* 2001;85(1):92-93.

[71]  Kandzari DE, Berger PB, Kastrati A, Steinhubl SR, Mehilli J, Dotzer F, Ten
      Berg JM, Neumann FJ, Bollwein H, Dirschinger J, Schomig A. Influence of
      treatment duration with a 600-mg dose of clopidogrel before percutaneous
      coronary revascularization. *J Am Coll Cardiol.* 2004;44(11):2133-2136.

[72]  Patti G, Colonna G, Pasceri V, Pepe LL, Montinaro A, Di Sciascio G.
      Randomized trial of high loading dose of clopidogrel for reduction of
      periprocedural myocardial infarction in patients undergoing coronary
      intervention: results from the ARMYDA-2 (Antiplatelet therapy for
      Reduction of MYocardial Damage during Angioplasty) study. *Circulation.*
      2005;111(16):2099-2106.

[73]  von Beckerath N, Taubert D, Pogatsa-Murray G, Schomig E, Kastrati A,
      Schomig A. Absorption, metabolization, and antiplatelet effects of 300-,
      600-, and 900-mg loading doses of clopidogrel: results of the ISAR-
      CHOICE (Intracoronary Stenting and Antithrombotic Regimen: Choose
      Between 3 High Oral Doses for Immediate Clopidogrel Effect) Trial.
      *Circulation.* 2005;112(19):2946-2950.

[74]  Montalescot G, Sideris G, Meuleman C, Bal-dit-Sollier C, Lellouche N,
      Steg PG, Slama M, Milleron O, Collet JP, Henry P, Beygui F, Drouet L. A
      randomized comparison of high clopidogrel loading doses in patients with
      non-ST-segment elevation acute coronary syndromes: the ALBION
      (Assessment of the Best Loading Dose of Clopidogrel to Blunt Platelet
      Activation, Inflammation and Ongoing Necrosis) trial. *J Am Coll Cardiol.*
      2006;48(5):931-938.

[75]  Van de Werf F, Bax J, Betriu A, Blomstrom-Lundqvist C, Crea F, Falk V,
      Filippatos G, Fox K, Huber K, Kastrati A, Rosengren A, Steg PG, Tubaro
      M, Verheugt F, Weidinger F, Weis M, Vahanian A, Camm J, De Caterina R,
      Dean V, Dickstein K, Funck-Brentano C, Hellemans I, Kristensen SD,
      McGregor K, Sechtem U, Silber S, Tendera M, Widimsky P, Zamorano JL,
      Aguirre FV, Al-Attar N, Alegria E, Andreotti F, Benzer W, Breithardt O,
      Danchin N, Di Mario C, Dudek D, Gulba D, Halvorsen S, Kaufmann P,
      Kornowski R, Lip GY, Rutten F. Management of acute myocardial
      infarction in patients presenting with persistent ST-segment elevation: the
      Task Force on the Management of ST-Segment Elevation Acute Myocardial
      Infarction of the European Society of Cardiology. *Eur Heart J.*
      2008;29(23):2909-2945.

[76]  Kushner FG, Hand M, Smith SC, Jr., King SB, 3rd, Anderson JL, Antman
      EM, Bailey SR, Bates ER, Blankenship JC, Casey DE, Jr., Green LA,
      Hochman JS, Jacobs AK, Krumholz HM, Morrison DA, Ornato JP, Pearle
      DL, Peterson ED, Sloan MA, Whitlow PL, Williams DO. 2009 Focused
      Updates: ACC/AHA Guidelines for the Management of Patients With ST-
      Elevation Myocardial Infarction (updating the 2004 Guideline and 2007

Focused Update) and ACC/AHA/SCAI Guidelines on Percutaneous Coronary Intervention (updating the 2005 Guideline and 2007 Focused Update): a report of the American College of Cardiology Foundation/American Heart Association Task Force on Practice Guidelines. *Circulation.* 2009;120(22):2271-2306.

[77] Angiolillo DJ, Shoemaker SB, Desai B, Yuan H, Charlton RK, Bernardo E, Zenni MM, Guzman LA, Bass TA, Costa MA. Randomized comparison of a high clopidogrel maintenance dose in patients with diabetes mellitus and coronary artery disease: results of the Optimizing Antiplatelet Therapy in Diabetes Mellitus (OPTIMUS) study. *Circulation.* 2007;115(6):708-716.

[78] von Beckerath N, Kastrati A, Wieczorek A, Pogatsa-Murray G, Sibbing D, Graf I, Schomig A. A double-blind, randomized study on platelet aggregation in patients treated with a daily dose of 150 or 75 mg of clopidogrel for 30 days. *Eur Heart J.* 2007;28(15):1814-1819.

[79] Neubauer H, Lask S, Engelhardt A, Mugge A. How to optimise clopidogrel therapy? Reducing the low-response incidence by aggregometry-guided therapy modification. *Thromb Haemost.* 2008;99(2):357-362.

[80] Bonello L, Camoin-Jau L, Arques S, Boyer C, Panagides D, Wittenberg O, Simeoni MC, Barragan P, Dignat-George F, Paganelli F. Adjusted clopidogrel loading doses according to vasodilator-stimulated phosphoprotein phosphorylation index decrease rate of major adverse cardiovascular events in patients with clopidogrel resistance: a multicenter randomized prospective study. *J Am Coll Cardiol.* 2008;51(14):1404-1411.

[81] Marcucci R, Gori AM, Paniccia R, Giusti B, Valente S, Giglioli C, Buonamici P, Antoniucci D, Abbate R, Gensini GF. Cardiovascular death and nonfatal myocardial infarction in acute coronary syndrome patients receiving coronary stenting are predicted by residual platelet reactivity to ADP detected by a point-of-care assay: a 12-month follow-up. *Circulation.* 2009;119(2):237-242.

[82] Price MJ, Endemann S, Gollapudi RR, Valencia R, Stinis CT, Levisay JP, Ernst A, Sawhney NS, Schatz RA, Teirstein PS. Prognostic significance of post-clopidogrel platelet reactivity assessed by a point-of-care assay on thrombotic events after drug-eluting stent implantation. *Eur Heart J.* 2008;29(8):992-1000.

[83] Kuliczkowski W, Witkowski A, Polonski L, Watala C, Filipiak K, Budaj A, Golanski J, Sitkiewicz D, Pregowski J, Gorski J, Zembala M, Opolski G, Huber K, Arnesen H, Kristensen SD, De Caterina R. Interindividual variability in the response to oral antiplatelet drugs: a position paper of the Working Group on antiplatelet drugs resistance appointed by the Section of Cardiovascular Interventions of the Polish Cardiac Society, endorsed by the

Working Group on Thrombosis of the European Society of Cardiology. *Eur Heart J.* 2009;30(4):426-435.

[84]   Wallentin L, Varenhorst C, James S, Erlinge D, Braun OO, Jakubowski JA, Sugidachi A, Winters KJ, Siegbahn A. Prasugrel achieves greater and faster P2Y12receptor-mediated platelet inhibition than clopidogrel due to more efficient generation of its active metabolite in aspirin-treated patients with coronary artery disease. *Eur Heart J.* 2008;29(1):21-30.

[85]   Wiviott SD, Trenk D, Frelinger AL, O'Donoghue M, Neumann FJ, Michelson AD, Angiolillo DJ, Hod H, Montalescot G, Miller DL, Jakubowski JA, Cairns R, Murphy SA, McCabe CH, Antman EM, Braunwald E. Prasugrel compared with high loading- and maintenance-dose clopidogrel in patients with planned percutaneous coronary intervention: the Prasugrel in Comparison to Clopidogrel for Inhibition of Platelet Activation and Aggregation-Thrombolysis in Myocardial Infarction 44 trial. *Circulation.* 2007;116(25):2923-2932.

[86]   Wiviott SD, Braunwald E, McCabe CH, Montalescot G, Ruzyllo W, Gottlieb S, Neumann FJ, Ardissino D, De Servi S, Murphy SA, Riesmeyer J, Weerakkody G, Gibson CM, Antman EM. Prasugrel versus clopidogrel in patients with acute coronary syndromes. *N Engl J Med.* 2007;357(20):2001-2015.

[87]   Wiviott SD, Braunwald E, Angiolillo DJ, Meisel S, Dalby AJ, Verheugt FW, Goodman SG, Corbalan R, Purdy DA, Murphy SA, McCabe CII, Antman EM. Greater clinical benefit of more intensive oral antiplatelet therapy with prasugrel in patients with diabetes mellitus in the trial to assess improvement in therapeutic outcomes by optimizing platelet inhibition with prasugrel-Thrombolysis in Myocardial Infarction 38. *Circulation.* 2008;118(16):1626-1636.

[88]   Husted S, Emanuelsson H, Heptinstall S, Sandset PM, Wickens M, Peters G. Pharmacodynamics, pharmacokinetics, and safety of the oral reversible P2Y12 antagonist AZD6140 with aspirin in patients with atherosclerosis: a double-blind comparison to clopidogrel with aspirin. *Eur Heart J.* 2006;27(9):1038-1047.

[89]   Cannon CP, Husted S, Harrington RA, Scirica BM, Emanuelsson H, Peters G, Storey RF. Safety, tolerability, and initial efficacy of AZD6140, the first reversible oral adenosine diphosphate receptor antagonist, compared with clopidogrel, in patients with non-ST-segment elevation acute coronary syndrome: primary results of the DISPERSE-2 trial. *J Am Coll Cardiol.* 2007;50(19):1844-1851.

[90]   Wallentin L, Becker RC, Budaj A, Cannon CP, Emanuelsson H, Held C, Horrow J, Husted S, James S, Katus H, Mahaffey KW, Scirica BM, Skene A, Steg PG, Storey RF, Harrington RA, Freij A, Thorsen M. Ticagrelor

versus clopidogrel in patients with acute coronary syndromes. *N Engl J Med.* 2009;361(11):1045-1057.

[91] Cannon CP, Harrington RA, James S, Ardissino D, Becker RC, Emanuelsson H, Husted S, Katus H, Keltai M, Khurmi NS, Kontny F, Lewis BS, Steg PG, Storey RF, Wojdyla D, Wallentin L. Comparison of ticagrelor with clopidogrel in patients with a planned invasive strategy for acute coronary syndromes (PLATO): a randomised double-blind study. *Lancet.*375(9711):283-293.

[92] Steg PG. STEMI subanalysis of the PLATO trial. Paper presented at: American Heart Association 2009 Scientific Sessions November 15th 2009, 2010; Orland, Florida, USA.

[93] Gurbel PA, Bliden KP, Butler K, Tantry US, Gesheff T, Wei C, Teng R, Antonino MJ, Patil SB, Karunakaran A, Kereiakes DJ, Parris C, Purdy D, Wilson V, Ledley GS, Storey RF. Randomized double-blind assessment of the ONSET and OFFSET of the antiplatelet effects of ticagrelor versus clopidogrel in patients with stable coronary artery disease: the ONSET/OFFSET study. *Circulation.* 2009;120(25):2577-2585.

[94] Gurbel PA, Bliden KP, Butler K, Antonino MJ, Wei C, Teng R, Rasmussen L, Storey RF, Nielsen T, Eikelboom JW, Sabe-Affaki G, Husted S, Kereiakes DJ, Henderson D, Patel DV, Tantry US. Response to Ticagrelor in Clopidogrel Nonresponders and Responders and Effect of Switching Therapies: The RESPOND Study. *Circulation.*121(10):1188-1199.

[95] Greenbaum AB, Grines CL, Bittl JA, Becker RC, Kereiakes DJ, Gilchrist IC, Clegg J, Stankowski JE, Grogan DR, Harrington RA, Emanuelsson H, Weaver WD. Initial experience with an intravenous P2Y12 platelet receptor antagonist in patients undergoing percutaneous coronary intervention: results from a 2-part, phase II, multicenter, randomized, placebo- and active-controlled trial. *Am Heart J.* 2006;151(3):689 e681-689 e610.

[96] Bhatt DL, Lincoff AM, Gibson CM, Stone GW, McNulty S, Montalescot G, Kleiman NS, Goodman SG, White HD, Mahaffey KW, Pollack CV, Jr., Manoukian SV, Widimsky P, Chew DP, Cura F, Manukov I, Tousek F, Jafar MZ, Arneja J, Skerjanec S, Harrington RA. Intravenous platelet blockade with cangrelor during PCI. *N Engl J Med.* 2009;361(24):2330-2341.

[97] Harrington RA, Stone GW, McNulty S, White HD, Lincoff AM, Gibson CM, Pollack CV, Jr., Montalescot G, Mahaffey KW, Kleiman NS, Goodman SG, Amine M, Angiolillo DJ, Becker RC, Chew DP, French WJ, Leisch F, Parikh KH, Skerjanec S, Bhatt DL. Platelet inhibition with cangrelor in patients undergoing PCI. *N Engl J Med.* 2009;361(24):2318-2329.

# Index

trial, 10, 21, 22, 23, 26, 27, 28, 29, 31, 33, 34, 37, 41, 43, 44

## U

uniform, 29
unstable angina, 1, 27, 36
updating, 41
uric acid, 28

## V

Valencia, 42
variations, 35
vasodilator, 10, 42

## W

withdrawal, 19